CW00417953

Vasculitis Symptoms

Chapter List:

Book Introduction:

Within the intricate network of human veins lies a mysterious adversary that affects countless lives – Vasculitis. In "Journey Through the Veins:

Navigating the Depths of Vasculitis," we embark on an emotional expedition, delving into the intricate world of this complex and often enigmatic disease.

Vasculitis, an inflammation of blood vessels, emerges as a silent intruder, striking people of all ages and backgrounds, leaving no one untouched. This book serves as a guiding light, illuminating the path for patients, caregivers, and medical professionals to understand and navigate the challenges posed by Vasculitis.

In this comprehensive guide, we traverse the depths of Vasculitis, unraveling its intricacies, and shedding light on its elusive nature. Each chapter acts as a milestone on this transformative journey, providing invaluable knowledge, heartfelt stories, and empowering strategies.

From the initial signs that whisper its arrival to the arduous path of diagnosis and treatment, we explore the diverse manifestations of Vasculitis in different organ systems. By interweaving scientific insights, personal anecdotes, and emotional narratives, this book aims to create a profound connection, resonating with the readers on a deeply human level.

As we venture into the realm of Vasculitis, we encounter remarkable individuals who embody resilience, courage, and unwavering determination. Their stories become beacons of hope, inspiring others to navigate their own paths with strength and grace. Additionally, we examine the latest advancements in research, shining a ray of hope on the horizon for a brighter future.

Ultimately, "Journey Through the Veins: Navigating the Depths of

Vasculitis" is more than just a book – it is a lifeline for those battling Vasculitis, a compass guiding them through the darkest hours. With empathy as our compass, knowledge as our fuel, and the shared human experience as our guide, let us embark on this profound expedition together.

Chapter 1: Unraveling the Enigma: Introduction to Vasculitis

Within the intricate tapestry of human health, a silent enigma lurks: Vasculitis. In this opening chapter, we embark on a journey of discovery, unraveling the intricate nature of this perplexing condition. Vasculitis, as the name suggests, involves inflammation of the blood vessels—a complex web that connects our entire body. But what triggers this intricate network to turn against us

We delve into the origins of Vasculitis, exploring potential causes and risk factors that contribute to its development. From genetic predispositions to environmental triggers, we navigate the labyrinth of possibilities, seeking to understand why and how this enigmatic disease takes hold.

Through personal stories, medical insights, and compelling research, we shed light on the diverse manifestations of Vasculitis. As we peel back the layers, we uncover the telltale signs and symptoms that herald the presence of this stealthy intruder.

Join us as we embark on a quest for knowledge and understanding, eager to unravel the enigma that is Vasculitis. Together, we shall navigate the depths of this intricate condition, empowering ourselves with the insights needed to confront the challenges that lie ahead.

Chapter 2: The Silent Intruder: Understanding Vasculitis Causes

In the shadows of our lives, an invisible adversary lurks, wreaking havoc on our very core. Vasculitis, the silent intruder, strikes without warning, disrupting the delicate balance within our bodies. In this chapter, we embark on a poignant exploration, seeking to understand the causes that give rise to this formidable enemy.

As we delve deeper into the realms of Vasculitis, we encounter a myriad of triggers, each capable of awakening the dormant beast within. Environmental factors, infections, and even medications can all conspire to set off a cascade of events, igniting the flames of inflammation within our vulnerable vessels.

Yet, the mystery remains unsolved. Why do some fall victim to this insidious foe while others escape unscathed Genetics intertwine with fate, as we uncover the intricate dance between our DNA and the forces that shape our lives. Through tales of genetic predisposition and familial connections, we witness the intricate tapestry of hereditary influences in Vasculitis.

But it is not merely a matter of genes and chance. Our surroundings hold secrets of their own. Toxins in the air we breathe, the food we consume, and the chemicals we encounter may leave an indelible mark, triggering an immune system response that spirals out of control. The echoes of environmental factors resonate, urging us to take heed of the world we inhabit and its potential impact on our well-being.

As we navigate the labyrinthine corridors of Vasculitis causes, we confront the profound questions that arise. Why must some bear the burden of this silent intruder, while others remain untouched There are no easy answers, only the weight of uncertainty and the ache of uncharted territories.

Yet, amidst the darkness, a flicker of hope emerges. Research and medical advancements illuminate the path, guiding us toward a deeper understanding of this relentless foe. Through the power of knowledge, we find solace in the shared experiences of those who have walked this treacherous path before us.

Together, we stand, united in our quest for comprehension and armed with the resolve to face the challenges that lie ahead. Let us unravel the enigma of Vasculitis causes, not merely as observers but as warriors of empathy and champions of compassion. For within the depths of our collective journey, we uncover the strength to overcome, to fight, and to find healing amidst the tumultuous currents of Vasculitis.

Chapter 3: Signs in the Shadows: Early Warning Signs of Vasculitis

In the labyrinth of our bodies, Vasculitis weaves its intricate web, its presence often obscured, its signs concealed within the shadows. This chapter serves as a poignant guide, illuminating the early warning signs that whisper of its arrival. For in the realm of Vasculitis, knowledge becomes a shield, and awareness becomes a lifeline.

As we embark on this emotional expedition, we bear witness to the stories of those who have stood on the precipice of uncertainty. They recount the moments when the first ripples of Vasculitis made themselves known—subtle whispers of discomfort, fleeting sensations that hinted at a storm brewing beneath the surface.

Fatigue, like a heavy shroud, descends upon the weary, draining their vitality and clouding their days. Joint pain, like a persistent ache, steals away the joy of movement, leaving behind a trail of stiffness and immobility. Skin rashes, like silent messengers, paint a portrait of inflammation, a vivid reminder of the battle raging within.

But it is not only the physical realm that bears the marks of this unseen assailant. The heart, burdened with the weight of Vasculitis, may falter, its rhythm disrupted by the inflammation that knows no boundaries. The lungs, gasping for air, bear witness to the impact on the respiratory system, while the eyes, windows to the soul, may reveal the telltale signs of ocular Vasculitis.

With every symptom shared, a surge of recognition reverberates through the pages of this chapter. The sense of isolation, the fear of the unknown—these emotions find solace in the acknowledgement of shared experiences. And within this solidarity, a glimmer of hope emerges, promising that no one walks this path alone.

Through the collaborative efforts of medical professionals, we unravel the complexity of diagnosing Vasculitis.

We explore the intricate dance of medical testing, where blood work, biopsies, and imaging become the tools to decipher the enigma. Yet, we also acknowledge the challenges and uncertainties, the moments when the answers elude us, leaving us adrift in a sea of unanswered questions.

But even in the face of uncertainty, resilience prevails. We find strength in the stories of those who have confronted the early signs, who have faced the unknown with unwavering determination. Their journeys, interwoven with empathy and compassion, remind us that even amidst the shadows, there is light to be found.

In this chapter, we embrace the power of awareness. We heed the whispers, the subtle signs that beckon us to action. Armed with knowledge, we empower ourselves and others to seek answers, to advocate for our own well-being, and to navigate the labyrinthine path of early Vasculitis detection.

For within the shadows, a spark of hope ignites. Together, we shall cast a light on the signs in the darkness, illuminating the way forward and standing united against the silent intruder that is Vasculitis.

Chapter 4: Battling the Unknown: Diagnosis and Medical Testing for Vasculitis

In the battle against the unknown, we arm ourselves with courage and resolve, facing the daunting task of diagnosing Vasculitis head-on. This chapter is a testament to the relentless pursuit of answers, a heartfelt exploration of the medical tests and procedures that illuminate the path toward understanding.

Within the halls of hospitals and clinics, a symphony of technology and expertise intertwines, each note harmonizing with the next, striving to unravel the complexities of Vasculitis. Blood samples are taken, like threads of life, revealing the secrets hidden within. Laboratory analyses become a language of their own, translating the whispers of inflammation into tangible data.

Biopsies, a testament to resilience, extract fragments of tissue, guiding us toward the heart of the matter. Under the microscope's watchful eye, these delicate specimens become windows into the world of Vasculitis, offering glimpses of its destructive force.

Radiological imaging, a visual tapestry of our internal landscapes, uncovers the footprints of Vasculitis. X-rays, CT scans, and MRIs capture the invisible battle, revealing the ravages within our veins, our organs, our very being. Like cartographers, we map the terrain of this intricate disease, piecing together the puzzle with each image obtained.

Yet, the path to diagnosis is often paved with uncertainty and frustration. The road is winding, and the signs may be elusive, leaving many to wander in a labyrinth of unanswered questions. Misdiagnoses and misunderstandings become unwelcome companions, casting shadows of doubt upon the journey.

But through the tears of frustration, hope shines through. For within the medical community, there are dedicated healers who become guides and allies, their empathy and expertise lighting the way forward. They listen intently to the stories of patients, attuned to the nuances that may hold the key to unlocking the mysteries of Vasculitis.

Together, patient and physician navigate this uncharted territory, a partnership rooted in trust and shared purpose. The bond formed in these moments becomes a lifeline, fostering resilience and nurturing the seeds of healing.

In this chapter, we bear witness to the triumphs and tribulations that accompany the quest for a Vasculitis diagnosis. We stand alongside those who have weathered the storm, their stories testaments to the resilience of the human spirit. Through their experiences, we find solace, knowing that we are not alone in our struggle.

Armed with knowledge and the unwavering spirit of advocacy, we forge ahead, shining a light on the path less traveled. For within the labyrinth of diagnosis, hope abounds. Let us embrace the power of medical testing and the collaboration between patients and healthcare professionals, as we navigate the stormy seas of Vasculitis, inching closer to understanding and healing.

Chapter 5: Warriors of Resilience: Stories of Vasculitis Patients

Amidst the battlefield of Vasculitis, a community of warriors emerges, their stories echoing with resilience, courage, and unwavering determination. In this chapter, we delve into the lives of these extraordinary individuals, who have faced the relentless challenges posed by Vasculitis with unwavering strength.

Each story is a tapestry woven with threads of hope, struggle, and triumph. We meet warriors of all ages and backgrounds, their voices resounding with authenticity and vulnerability. Through their , we bear witness to the raw emotions that accompany the Vasculitis journey—fear, frustration, and despair, but also resilience, hope, and the unwavering spirit to defy the odds.

These warriors share their darkest moments—the days when pain consumed their bodies, when fatigue weighed heavy upon their shoulders, and when the future seemed shrouded in uncertainty. We walk beside them as they navigate the labyrinthine path of diagnosis, encounter setbacks, and endure the grueling treatments that mark their battle against Vasculitis.

Yet, within these stories lies the undeniable power of the human spirit. We witness the triumphs, both big and small—the moments when a glimmer of light breaks through the darkest clouds. A remission achieved, a treatment milestone reached, or simply a day of respite from the relentless grip of Vasculitis—these victories become beacons of hope, igniting the flame of resilience within us all.

Through shared experiences, these warriors become pillars of support for one another. They offer solace, understanding, and a sense of belonging in a world that often fails to grasp the magnitude of their journey. Together, they create a tapestry of strength, woven through shared tears, shared laughter, and the unwavering support that only those who have walked a similar path can provide.

Their stories remind us that Vasculitis does not define them—it is but a chapter in their lives, albeit a challenging one. We witness their determination to reclaim their sense of self, their unwavering spirit to rise above the limitations imposed by this relentless adversary. They show us that while Vasculitis may leave scars, both seen and unseen, it cannot extinguish the flame of resilience that burns within.

In sharing these stories, we honor the warriors who have faced Vasculitis head-on. Their voices inspire us to advocate for awareness, understanding, and improved treatment options. They remind us that behind each diagnosis is a life, a unique story waiting to be heard.

Together, let us amplify their voices, weaving their narratives into the fabric of our collective consciousness. For within the stories of these warriors, we find solace, inspiration, and the unwavering belief that we can overcome the challenges posed by Vasculitis, united as a community of resilience and strength.

Chapter 6: The Web Within: How Vasculitis Affects Different Organ Systems

Vasculitis, like an insidious spider, weaves its intricate web throughout our bodies, affecting diverse organ systems with its relentless grasp. In this chapter, we embark on a poignant exploration, shining a light on the far-reaching impact of Vasculitis and the toll it takes on our physical well-being.

Our journey begins at the heart, the epicenter of our existence. We uncover the profound consequences of Vasculitis on the cardiovascular system, where inflamed vessels disrupt the rhythm of life itself. The echoes of chest pain, palpitations, and shortness of breath resound, reminders of the heart's relentless battle against the relentless intruder.

We then traverse the intricate network of veins and arteries, witnessing the havoc wreaked upon our circulatory system. From inflamed blood vessels in the limbs that rob us of mobility to the fragile vessels within the eyes that threaten our vision, we encounter the collateral damage left in Vasculitis's wake.

The respiratory system, the gateway to life-giving breath, becomes a battleground. Lungs scarred by inflammation struggle to deliver oxygen to our bodies, leaving us breathless and weary. The simple act of filling our lungs becomes a Herculean task, a reminder of the invisible chains that Vasculitis seeks to bind us with.

But the impact of Vasculitis extends beyond the physical realm. We delve into the intricate connections between inflammation and the mind, exploring the emotional and psychological toll it exacts. Anxiety, depression, and the weight of chronic illness become unwelcome companions, as the battle against Vasculitis seeps into the very fabric of our being.

Digestive woes become a common companion on this tumultuous journey. Inflamed vessels disrupt the delicate balance within our gastrointestinal system, causing pain, nausea, and loss of appetite. Our bodies, once temples of nourishment, become battlegrounds where the simplest act of eating becomes an act of defiance.

As we navigate the depths of Vasculitis's impact on different organ systems, we encounter the resiliency of the human spirit. We witness the unwavering determination of individuals who refuse to be defined by their condition, who rise above the challenges with indomitable strength.

In the face of these adversities, medical advancements become beacons of hope. We explore the innovative treatments and therapies that strive to tame the relentless forces of Vasculitis, providing respite and reclaiming moments of normalcy.

Through the stories of those who have traversed this treacherous terrain, we find solace and kinship. Their experiences remind us that while Vasculitis may leave scars, both seen and unseen, it cannot extinguish the fire that burns within us. Together, we forge a bond of empathy and compassion, united in our shared journey.

In this chapter, we honor the resilience of the human spirit. We shed light on the web that Vasculitis weaves within us, recognizing the profound impact it has on our physical, emotional, and psychological well-being. Through understanding and support, we stand as a community, committed to raising awareness, advocating for improved treatments, and offering a lifeline of empathy to those navigating the intricate web of Vasculitis.

Chapter 7: Unmasking the Enemy: Identifying Different Types of Vasculitis

In the realm of Vasculitis, an invisible enemy wears many masks, each concealing its unique form and characteristics. In this chapter, we embark on an emotional journey of unmasking, seeking to identify the different types of Vasculitis that silently lurk within our veins.

As we lift the veil of ambiguity, we encounter a diverse cast of Vasculitis variants, each with its own distinctive traits and patterns. Giant Cell Arteritis, like a stealthy predator, targets the head and neck, its presence marked by throbbing headaches and tender scalp. Takayasu's Arteritis, an elusive foe, takes aim at the large arteries, hindering blood flow to vital organs and extremities.

Microscopic Polyangiitis, a silent infiltrator, attacks small blood vessels throughout the body, leaving behind a trail of systemic damage. Behçet's Disease, a master of disguise, unveils itself through a myriad of symptoms, from oral and genital ulcers to skin lesions and eye inflammation. These are but a few of the many faces that Vasculitis wears.

With each unveiling, we bear witness to the personal stories of those living with these distinct types of Vasculitis. They recount the moments when their lives were forever altered, when their bodies became battlegrounds, and their identities intertwined with the disease. Their narratives embody the courage and resilience needed to confront the unknown.

We navigate the complexities of diagnosis, where medical professionals wield their expertise to unravel the puzzle of Vasculitis subtypes. Biopsies, laboratory tests, and imaging studies become tools of detection, helping to decipher the specific variant that lies beneath the surface. Yet, we also acknowledge the challenges of misdiagnosis and the long and winding road to finding answers.

But in the face of adversity, hope prevails. We explore the advancements in medical research that shed light on the intricate nature of each Vasculitis type. Through international collaborations and dedicated scientists, we inch closer to unraveling the mysteries of these formidable adversaries. We celebrate the strides made in understanding the genetic, immunological, and environmental factors that contribute to their development.

Within the tapestry of unmasking, we find solidarity and shared experiences. The stories of those who have faced different types of Vasculitis become beacons of empathy, reminding us that we are not alone in our battles. In their voices, we discover a symphony of resilience, inspiring us to advocate for awareness, support, and improved treatment options.

Together, let us continue to unmask the enemy, to shed light on the different types of Vasculitis that pervade our lives. Through understanding, compassion, and the power of collective knowledge, we empower ourselves and one another to face these invisible adversaries head-on. For within the realm of unmasking, we find strength, unity, and the unwavering spirit to forge ahead on our Vasculitis journey.

Chapter 8: Armoring Our Defenses: Treatment Options for Vasculitis

In the battle against Vasculitis, we don our armor of hope and resilience, armed with a formidable arsenal of treatment options. This chapter delves into the emotional landscape of therapeutic strategies, exploring the ways in which we fortify our bodies and minds against the relentless onslaught of this complex disease.

Medical advancements have gifted us with an array of weapons to combat Vasculitis, each tailored to the unique characteristics of the enemy we face. Corticosteroids, like mighty shields, temper the flames of inflammation, offering respite and relief to those caught in the throes of the battle. Immunosuppressants, warriors of balance, work hand in hand to quell the overactive immune response, restoring harmony within our bodies.

But the path to treatment is not without its challenges. We navigate the delicate balance of managing side effects, the toll they take on our physical and emotional well-being. Yet, within these trials, a tapestry of resilience emerges as we adapt, seeking the best course of action to strike back against Vasculitis.

Biologic therapies, like arrows guided by precision, target the specific components of the immune system responsible for the relentless attacks. They offer a glimmer of hope, a ray of light in the face of adversity. We witness their transformative impact, the lives they have touched, and the promise they hold for a brighter future.

Yet, treatment extends beyond the physical realm. It encompasses the nurturing of our mental and emotional well-being, for the battles fought within the mind are just as crucial. Support networks, therapists, and the power of self-care become our allies, guiding us through the emotional turbulence that accompanies Vasculitis.

Within these pages, we encounter the stories of warriors who have faced the daunting task of treatment with unwavering strength. They share the highs and lows, the triumphs and setbacks that mark their journeys. Their narratives weave a tapestry of resilience, reminding us that even amidst the darkest moments, hope flickers like an eternal flame.

In the quest for effective treatment, we celebrate the collaborative efforts of medical professionals and researchers. We honor their tireless dedication to unraveling the complexities of Vasculitis, their unwavering commitment to improving the lives of those affected. Through their endeavors, the horizon of possibility expands, and new avenues of treatment emerge.

Together, we stand as advocates and champions, lifting our voices in unison. We call for increased awareness, improved access to care, and continued research. In the face of Vasculitis, we draw strength from the collective spirit of the community, forging ahead with determination and resilience.

In this chapter, we embrace the emotional terrain of treatment. We honor the choices made, the sacrifices endured, and the indomitable spirit that propels us forward. With each step, we inch closer to victory, building a future where Vasculitis is tamed, where treatment options abound, and where hope reigns supreme.

Chapter 9: Empowering the Self: Lifestyle Changes and Coping Strategies

In the face of Vasculitis's relentless presence, we don the armor of empowerment, seeking solace and strength within ourselves. This chapter is a testament to the transformative power of lifestyle changes and coping strategies, guiding us toward a path of resilience and inner healing.

Vasculitis demands that we adapt, that we forge a new relationship with our bodies and minds. We embark on a journey of self-discovery, exploring the profound impact of lifestyle choices on our well-being. From the nourishment we provide our bodies through mindful nutrition to the revitalizing power of exercise, we cultivate a sanctuary of self-care.

Diet becomes a powerful ally in our battle against Vasculitis, as we nourish our bodies with foods that promote healing and reduce inflammation. We uncover the therapeutic potential of vibrant fruits and vegetables, the anti-inflammatory properties of omega-3 fatty acids, and the delicate balance of nutrients that strengthen our immune systems.

Exercise becomes a testament to the resilience of the human spirit. We witness the transformative power of movement, as it releases endorphins and boosts our mental well-being. From gentle stretches that awaken our bodies to invigorating activities that challenge our limits, we embrace the healing potential that lies within.

But Vasculitis demands more than physical changes. It penetrates the very core of our emotional well-being. In the face of its tumultuous waves, we cultivate coping strategies that become lifelines of stability and strength. Mindfulness, meditation, and the healing power of art and music become our allies, grounding us amidst the storm.

Support networks, both online and offline, become pillars of strength, connecting us with others who understand our journey. In shared experiences, we find solace, validation, and the invaluable sense of community. The bonds we form become woven into the tapestry of our resilience, reminding us that we are not alone in this fight.

Within these pages, we encounter the stories of individuals who have embraced lifestyle changes and coping strategies as pillars of their resilience. Their narratives bear witness to the transformative power of self-empowerment, inspiring us to seek our own paths of healing and growth.

But this chapter also acknowledges the challenges and setbacks we may encounter along the way. Vasculitis tests our resolve, and there may be moments of frustration, grief, and exhaustion. In these moments, we draw strength from our collective experiences, knowing that we have the power to rise above the obstacles that lie before us.

Together, let us embrace the power of lifestyle changes and coping strategies, fostering a sense of empowerment within ourselves. Through self-care and self-compassion, we forge a sanctuary of healing amidst the chaos. We navigate the depths of Vasculitis, armed with resilience, and anchored in the belief that within us lies the power to thrive, to flourish, and to reclaim our lives.

In this chapter, we honor the transformative journey of self-empowerment. We celebrate the strength that resides within us all, urging us to embrace lifestyle changes, cultivate coping strategies, and find solace in the empowering realization that we hold the key to our own well-being.

Chapter 10: Allies in the Journey: Support and Resources for Vasculitis Patients

In the labyrinth of Vasculitis, we are not alone. This chapter is a heartfelt exploration of the allies who walk alongside us on this challenging journey. It is a testament to the power of support and the vast resources that exist to uplift and guide us through the labyrinthine path of Vasculitis.

Within the embrace of the Vasculitis community, we find solace and understanding. Support groups, both in-person and online, become sanctuaries of empathy, where shared experiences intertwine and bonds are forged. In the comforting of fellow warriors, we discover the strength to face the challenges that Vasculitis presents.

Medical professionals, beacons of expertise and compassion, become our allies in the battle against Vasculitis. From rheumatologists to specialized nurses, they provide guidance, knowledge, and a compassionate touch. Their unwavering dedication to our well-being becomes a lifeline, a source of hope and encouragement.

Patient advocacy organizations become beacons of light, tirelessly working to raise awareness, advocate for improved care, and foster connections within the Vasculitis community. They offer a wealth of resources, from educational materials to support networks, guiding us through the labyrinth of Vasculitis with expertise and compassion.

Research institutions and clinical trials pave the way toward a brighter future. Dedicated scientists and researchers devote their efforts to unraveling the mysteries of Vasculitis, seeking improved treatments and, ultimately, a cure. Their unwavering commitment becomes a source of inspiration, fueling our hope and optimism.

The power of storytelling emerges as a profound ally on our Vasculitis journey. Memoirs, articles, and personal narratives become windows into the lives of those who have walked this path before us. Through their , we find solace, guidance, and the courage to persevere.

Within the labyrinth, family and friends become pillars of unwavering support. Their love, patience, and understanding provide us with a sense of belonging, grounding us amidst the storm. Their presence becomes a constant reminder that we are not defined by our illness, but by the connections we foster and the love we share.

This chapter celebrates the allies who navigate the Vasculitis journey with us. We honor the strength and resilience of the community that surrounds us, urging us to reach out, to embrace the support that is offered, and to extend our own hand to those who may need it.

Let us stand together, united in our quest for understanding, compassion, and improved care. Let us recognize the power of support and resources in empowering us to face Vasculitis head-on. For within the collective strength of our allies lies the unwavering belief that we are not alone, that our voices matter, and that together, we can create a brighter future amidst the challenges of Vasculitis.

Chapter 11: Beyond the Physical: Emotional and Psychological Impact of Vasculitis

Vasculitis, like a tempest, not only ravages our bodies but also leaves an indelible mark on our emotional and psychological well-being. In this chapter, we delve into the depths of the emotional landscape, exploring the profound impact of Vasculitis on our inner selves.

The journey through Vasculitis is fraught with emotional turbulence. Fear, anxiety, and uncertainty become unwelcome companions, weaving their way into the fabric of our daily lives. The weight of chronic illness bears down upon us, casting shadows of doubt and vulnerability. Yet, within these shadows, glimmers of resilience emerge.

We confront the grief and loss that accompany the Vasculitis journey. The loss of our sense of invincibility, the loss of the life we once knew, and sometimes, the loss of our own identity. We mourn the dreams and aspirations that may have been altered by the relentless presence of this disease. Yet, amidst the grief, we find the seeds of transformation, the opportunity for growth and self-discovery.

Isolation can become an unwelcome companion, as the world around us may struggle to comprehend the invisible battles we face. We yearn for understanding, for validation, and for the reassurance that we are not alone. It is within the embrace of the Vasculitis community that we find solace—a sanctuary where empathy flows freely, where our experiences are acknowledged and shared.

The psychological impact of Vasculitis cannot be understated. Depression, anxiety, and mood disorders can intertwine with the physical manifestations of the disease, creating a complex web that demands our attention. Yet, within this web, we discover the resilience of the human spirit—the capacity to find strength in vulnerability and the power to rise above the challenges that confront us.

Professional support becomes a vital component of our emotional well-being. Therapists, counselors, and psychologists become guides, offering a safe space to explore the emotional intricacies of the Vasculitis journey. They provide the tools to navigate the storms, empowering us to build resilience and cultivate self-compassion.

But amidst the emotional landscape, there is also hope. We witness the transformative power of resilience—the ability to find beauty in the midst of adversity, to cherish the present moment, and to nurture gratitude for the strength we possess. Through art, writing, music, and other creative outlets, we discover the healing potential of self-expression.

In this chapter, we honor the emotional and psychological impact of Vasculitis. We acknowledge the complexities, the challenges, and the triumphs that shape our inner selves. Let us hold space for our emotions, embracing vulnerability as a testament to our humanity. Together, we stand, reminding one another that even amidst the storm, we possess the power to navigate the emotional landscape of Vasculitis with courage, grace, and unwavering hope.

Chapter 12: Illuminating Hope: Research and Breakthroughs in Vasculitis

In the realm of Vasculitis, hope shines as a guiding light, illuminating the path toward progress and breakthroughs. This chapter is a testament to the unwavering dedication of researchers and the transformative power of scientific advancements in the fight against Vasculitis.

Within the laboratories and research institutions, brilliant minds tirelessly work to unravel the intricate mysteries of Vasculitis. They strive to understand the underlying mechanisms, the genetic and environmental factors that contribute to its development. With each discovery, they inch closer to unraveling the enigma that shrouds this complex disease.

Clinical trials become beacons of hope, offering the possibility of new treatments and improved outcomes. They represent a bridge between scientific innovation and the individuals who bravely step forward to participate, lending their strength to the pursuit of knowledge. Through their participation, they become partners in the quest for a brighter future.

Through research, we gain a deeper understanding of the diverse subtypes of Vasculitis. We uncover the nuances that shape their clinical presentation, the specific markers that guide diagnosis and treatment. This knowledge becomes a powerful tool, empowering healthcare professionals to provide more accurate and personalized care.

Breakthroughs in treatment pave the way toward improved outcomes and quality of life for Vasculitis patients. Innovative therapies emerge, targeting the specific mechanisms of inflammation and immune dysregulation. These advancements offer the promise of better disease control, reduced side effects, and a brighter future for those living with Vasculitis.

But research goes beyond the realms of laboratory and clinical trials. It encompasses the power of collaboration, as experts from different fields join forces, pooling their knowledge and expertise. Within these collaborative endeavors, new perspectives emerge, and innovative solutions are born. The global Vasculitis community stands united, crossing borders and boundaries to drive progress forward.

In the wake of these advancements, hope flourishes. We witness the transformative impact they have on the lives of those living with Vasculitis. Remissions are achieved, relapses are reduced, and the burden of the disease is lightened. These victories become beacons of hope, shining a light on the path toward improved care and a brighter future.

In this chapter, we honor the resilience of the human spirit and the dedication of researchers who tirelessly strive to conquer Vasculitis. We celebrate the triumphs of scientific discovery and the breakthroughs that bring us closer to understanding and treating this complex disease.

Together, let us embrace the illumination of hope. Let us amplify the voices of researchers, advocates, and individuals living with Vasculitis, advocating for increased funding, support, and awareness. For within the realm of research and breakthroughs, lies the promise of a future where Vasculitis is tamed, where treatment options abound, and where hope reigns supreme.

Chapter 13: Embracing the Light: Finding Meaning and Purpose in the Vasculitis Journey

Within the intricate tapestry of the Vasculitis journey, we uncover the profound potential for finding meaning and purpose. This chapter is an emotional exploration of the transformative power that emerges when we embrace the light that shines amidst the challenges of living with Vasculitis.

In the depths of adversity, we embark on a journey of self-discovery, seeking to unearth the hidden gems of purpose that lie within us. We delve into the realms of our passions, our interests, and the unique gifts that make us who we are. In embracing these aspects of our identity, we reclaim a sense of self and find solace amidst the storm.

Living with Vasculitis grants us a unique perspective—an opportunity to cherish the simple joys, to find beauty in the smallest of moments. We learn to savor the warmth of a loved one's touch, the vibrant colors of nature, and the symphony of laughter that resounds within our lives. Through this newfound appreciation, we uncover a profound sense of gratitude and resilience.

Vasculitis becomes a catalyst for personal growth and transformation. We navigate the labyrinthine path, gaining insights and wisdom that shape our lives in unexpected ways. It challenges us to tap into our inner strength, to cultivate resilience and adaptability, and to embrace the ever-changing nature of our existence.

Within the Vasculitis community, we find inspiration and connection. We witness the power of support and empathy, as we come together to uplift and encourage one another. In sharing our stories, we inspire hope in others, forging bonds that transcend the boundaries of illness.

Through advocacy, we become agents of change. We raise our voices, speaking out for increased awareness, improved access to care, and research funding. We empower ourselves and others, ensuring that the experiences of those living with Vasculitis are heard and understood.

But perhaps the most profound aspect of finding meaning in the Vasculitis journey is the opportunity to make a difference in the lives of others. We become beacons of hope, extending a helping hand to those who walk a similar path. Through our experiences, we offer guidance, support, and a listening ear, nurturing a sense of belonging within the Vasculitis community.

In this chapter, we honor the transformative power of finding meaning and purpose amidst the challenges of Vasculitis. We celebrate the resilience, wisdom, and compassion that emerge when we embrace the light that shines within us. Let us continue to navigate the Vasculitis journey with open hearts, acknowledging the transformative potential that lies within, and spreading the radiance of hope to all who need it.

Together, we illuminate the path with our stories, our advocacy, and our unwavering spirit. For within the embrace of purpose and meaning, we discover that Vasculitis does not define us, but rather serves as a catalyst for growth, compassion, and the unyielding pursuit of a life lived with purpose and passion.

Chapter 14: The Light of Connection: Building Relationships in the Vasculitis Community

In the vast expanse of the Vasculitis journey, we discover the transformative power of connection. This chapter is a heartfelt exploration of the relationships that bloom within the Vasculitis community, illuminating our lives with empathy, support, and the unbreakable bonds that unite us.

Within the embrace of the Vasculitis community, we find solace and understanding that transcends . We connect with individuals who intimately comprehend the challenges we face, who walk alongside us on this winding path. In their presence, we discover the healing power of shared experiences and the comfort that comes from knowing we are not alone.

Friendships blossom, nourished by empathy, compassion, and a mutual understanding that extends beyond the confines of Vasculitis. We forge connections with individuals who become pillars of support, offering a steady hand to hold during the stormy moments. Together, we celebrate triumphs, lend a listening ear, and find strength in the unwavering bond that binds us.

Family members and loved ones become our steadfast allies, navigating

the intricacies of Vasculitis by our side.
Their love, patience, and unwavering
support become beacons of light,
illuminating our darkest moments.
They champion our resilience, uplift
our spirits, and remind us of the
unyielding strength we possess.

In the virtual realm, the Vasculitis
community becomes a tapestry woven
with threads of hope and unity. Online
support groups, forums, and social
media platforms offer spaces where
individuals can share their stories, seek
guidance, and offer of encouragement.
These digital connections transcend
distance, bridging the gaps between
continents, and fostering a sense of
global camaraderie.

Healthcare professionals become allies,
their expertise guiding us through the
complexities of Vasculitis. With their
knowledge and compassion, they
become trusted partners in our journey,

offering guidance, treatments, and a listening ear. Their presence provides reassurance that we are not alone in navigating the labyrinth of this complex disease.

Advocacy organizations stand as beacons of support and information, tirelessly working to raise awareness, promote research, and advocate for improved care. Through their efforts, they empower individuals living with Vasculitis, amplifying their voices and driving change. These organizations become a rallying point for the community, fostering unity and providing vital resources.

In this chapter, we honor the transformative power of connection within the Vasculitis community. We celebrate the relationships that uplift and inspire us, forging bonds that transcend the limitations imposed by illness. Together, we navigate the journey with hearts intertwined, reminding one another that we are stronger when we lean on each other.

Let us embrace the light of connection, extending our hands to those who seek solace and understanding. Through empathy, compassion, and shared experiences, we build a community that thrives on support and unity. In the Vasculitis community, we find strength, comfort, and the unwavering belief that together, we can conquer the challenges that lie before us.

With each connection we forge, we illuminate the path for others, guiding them toward the light of hope and understanding. For within the embrace of relationships, we discover that the Vasculitis journey, though challenging, is also a tapestry woven with compassion, resilience, and the transformative power of connection.

Chapter 15: The Light Within: Cultivating Resilience and Finding Hope

Amidst the tumultuous journey of Vasculitis, we discover an unwavering light that burns within us—the light of resilience and hope. In this final chapter, we delve into the depths of our inner strength, embracing the power that resides within, and finding hope in even the darkest of moments.

Resilience becomes our steadfast companion as we navigate the twists and turns of the Vasculitis journey. It is the unwavering spirit that propels us forward, even when the path seems insurmountable. It is the ability to adapt, to bounce back from setbacks, and to find meaning and purpose in the face of adversity.

Within the core of resilience lies the unbreakable flame of hope. It is the beacon that guides us through the darkest nights, reminding us that there is light at the end of the tunnel. It fuels our courage, our determination, and our belief that we have the strength to overcome the challenges that Vasculitis presents.

We find hope in the triumphs, both big and small—the moments of reprieve from pain, the remissions achieved, and the treatments that offer respite. We discover hope in the stories of those who have walked this path before us, witnessing their resilience and knowing that we too can persevere.

Even in the face of uncertainty, hope whispers to us that tomorrow holds the promise of new breakthroughs, improved treatments, and a brighter future. It emboldens us to dream, to set goals, and to live each day with intention and gratitude.

Cultivating hope becomes an active choice—a conscious decision to seek out the silver linings amidst the storm clouds. It is in the simple joys of everyday life—the warmth of a smile, the touch of a loved one's hand—that hope finds its roots and blossoms.

Through self-compassion, we nurture the light within. We extend kindness to ourselves, acknowledging the challenges we face and allowing space for healing and growth. We celebrate our resilience, our strength, and the battles we have fought with unwavering courage.

In the Vasculitis community, we find a wellspring of hope. We stand united, sharing our stories, our triumphs, and our vulnerabilities. We lift each other up, offering support, encouragement, and a reminder that we are not alone in this journey.

This final chapter serves as a testament to the power of resilience and hope in the face of Vasculitis. It honors the flame that burns within each of us, igniting our spirits, and reminding us of our inherent strength. Let us carry this light forward, sharing it with others who may need it, and fostering a community built on hope, compassion, and unwavering support.

Together, we stand as beacons of resilience and hope, illuminating the path for those who come after us. We forge ahead, guided by the light within, knowing that with each step we take, we are shaping a future where Vasculitis is understood, where treatments abound, and where hope shines eternally.

Printed in Great Britain
by Amazon

38512322R00036